INDIAN COOKBOOK
2021

DELICIOUS RECIPES FROM THE INDIAN TRADITION

SECOND EDITION

CHARLOTTE AHUJA

Table of Contents

Introduction

Indian food varies enormously. Whatever type of food you might be interested in – meat, fish or vegetarian – you will find a recipe to suit your palate and mood. While curry is inevitably associated with India, this term is simply used for meats or vegetables cooked in a spicy sauce, usually eaten with rice or Indian breads. As this collection of a thousand Indian recipes will show you, Indian food is not limited to the familiar restaurant favorites.

Food is taken very seriously in India and cooking is considered an art. Each Indian state has its own traditions, culture, lifestyle and food. Even individual households may have their own secret recipes for the powders and pastes that form the backbone of the dish. However, what all Indian dishes have in common is the delicate alchemy of spices that gives them their characteristic flavor.

The recipes in the book are authentic, such as you might encounter in an Indian home – yet they are simple, so if this is the first time that you are going to cook Indian food, relax. All you need to do is turn the pages, pick what tickles your fancy, and create a delicious meal, the Indian way!

Green Chilli Pickle

Ingredients

10 green chillies, slit

1 tsp salt

4 tsp ground mustard

1 tsp turmeric

Juice of 2 lemons

Method

- Mix all the ingredients together. Transfer the mixture to a clean, dry jar with a tight lid. Set aside for a day in a cool, dry place.

NOTE: *This can be stored in the refrigerator for a month.*

Sweet Tomato Chutney

Ingredients

2 tsp refined vegetable oil

4 dry red chillies

1 tsp turmeric

2.5cm/1in root ginger, chopped

4 tomatoes, chopped

125g/4½oz sugar

Salt to taste

Method

- Heat the oil in a saucepan. Add the chillies, turmeric and ginger. Fry on a medium heat for 1 minute. Add the remaining ingredients and cook the mixture until it is thick.
- Store in a clean, dry jar.

NOTE: *This can be stored for up to a month in the refrigerator.*

Apple Chutney

Ingredients

250g/9oz apples, peeled

120ml/4fl oz water

2 garlic cloves, crushed

2.5cm/1in root ginger, shredded

120ml/4fl oz malt vinegar

125g/4½oz sugar

Salt to taste

Method

- Slice the apples. Place in a saucepan with all the ingredients.
- Cook on a medium heat till tender.
- Cool and store in an airtight jar.

NOTE: *This can be stored for up to a week in the refrigerator.*

Bengali Mango Pickle

Ingredients

1 tsp salt

½ tsp turmeric

1 tsp chilli powder

150g/5½oz jaggery*

250g/9oz unripe mangoes, chopped into 2.5cm/1in pieces

2 tbsp mustard oil

2 tsp panch phoron*

4 red chillies, slit lengthways

Method

- Mix the salt, turmeric, chilli powder, jaggery and mangoes together. Set aside for 2 hours.
- Heat the oil in a saucepan. Add the panch phoron and the slit red chillies. Let them splutter for 15 seconds.
- Add the mango mixture. Cook on a low heat for 15 minutes, stirring occasionally, until the jaggery turns into a thick syrup.
- Remove from the heat and allow the mixture to cool. Store in a clean, dry jar.

NOTE: *This can be stored in a refrigerator for up to a week.*

Gujarati Sweet Mango Pickle

Ingredients

2 tsp salt

1 tsp turmeric

500g/1lb 2oz unripe mangoes, peeled and grated

400g/14oz sugar

1 tsp asafoetida

1 tbsp chilli powder

2 tsp ground cumin

Method

- Add salt and turmeric to the grated mangoes. Mix well and set aside for an hour.

- Add the sugar and cook the mixture in a sauepan on a low heat till the mixture has a consistency like maple syrup.
- Add the asafoetida, chilli powder and ground cumin. Mix well. Cook for another minute.
- Store in a clean, dry jar.

NOTE: *This can be stored in the refrigerator for a month.*

Ginger Pickle

Ingredients

250g/9oz root ginger, julienned

1 green chilli, finely chopped

3 tbsp refined vegetable oil

¾ tsp mustard seeds

8 curry leaves

1 dry red chilli

100g/3½oz tamarind paste

¼ tsp turmeric

¼ tsp chilli powder

125g/4½oz jaggery*, grated

1 tsp salt

60ml/2fl oz water

Method

- Fry the ginger and green chilli in 2 tbsp oil till brown. Set aside.
- Heat the remaining oil in a saucepan. Add the mustard seeds, curry leaves and red chilli. Let them splutter for 15 seconds.
- Add the fried ginger and green chilli mixture along with all the remaining ingredients. Simmer for 7-8 minutes. Cool and store in an airtight bottle.

NOTE: *This can be stored in the refrigerator for a fortnight.*

Pickled Chicken

Ingredients

1kg/2¼lb unripe chicken, chopped

250ml/8fl oz white vinegar

100ml/3½fl oz mustard oil

2 tsp ginger paste

2 tsp garlic paste

1½ tsp turmeric

1½ tsp chilli powder

2 tsp kalonji seeds*

3 black cardamom pods

8 cloves

Salt to taste

Method

- Mix the chicken with vinegar. Marinate for 3 hours. Pound and set aside.
- Heat the oil in a saucepan. Add the chicken mixture along with all the remaining ingredients. Simmer till the vinegar is absor bed.

NOTE: *This can be stored in the refrigerator for a month.*

Prawn Pickle

Ingredients

1 tsp turmeric

1 tsp chilli powder

1 tsp fenugreek seeds, ground

1 tsp mustard seeds, ground

Salt to taste

1 tbsp white vinegar

250g/9oz prawns, cleaned and de-veined

3 tbsp refined vegetable oil

¼ tsp mustard seeds

¼ tsp fenugreek seeds

¼ tsp asafoetida

Method

- Mix the turmeric, chilli powder, ground fenugreek, ground mustard and salt.
- Add this mixture, along with half the vinegar, to the prawns. Marinate for 2 hours.
- Heat the oil in a saucepan. Add the mustard seeds and fenugreek seeds. Let them splutter for 15 seconds.
- Add the asafoetida and the marinated punripens. Mix well.
- Cook on a low heat for 10 minutes.
- Add the remaining vinegar and continue to cook on a low heat for another 2-3 minutes.
- Remove from the heat and allow it to cool.
- Store in a clean, dry jar.

NOTE: *This can be stored in the refrigerator for a week.*

Onion Chutney

Ingredients

1 large onion, finely sliced

2 tbsp ready-made Indian mango pickle

1 small green chilli

Salt to taste

Method

- Pound all the ingredients into a thick paste.
- Store in a clean, dry jar.

NOTE: *This can be kept in the refrigerator for 2 days.*

Sweet & Sour Lime Pickle

Ingredients

500ml/16fl oz malt vinegar

1½ tsp salt

250ml/8fl oz water

10 large limes, quartered

1cm/½in root ginger, finely sliced

12 garlic cloves, finely sliced

5cm/2in cinnamon

8 cloves

375g/13oz sugar

Method

- Mix the vinegar, salt and half the water in a saucepan. Bring to a boil.
- Add the lime pieces, ginger, garlic, cinnamon and cloves. Cook for 7-8 minutes. Set aside.
- Melt the sugar in the remaining water and simmer till thick. Add the lime mixture. Mix well and remove from the heat.
- Cool and store in a clean, dry jar. Set aside for 3-4 days.

NOTE: *This can be stored in the refrigerator for a month.*

Turnip Pickle

Ingredients

250g/9oz turnips, chopped into 2.5cm/1in pieces

240ml/6fl oz water

120ml/¼fl oz refined vegetable oil

8 garlic cloves, crushed

1 tbsp ginger paste

240ml/6fl oz malt vinegar

125g/4½oz jaggery*,

grated

1 tsp chilli powder

4 cloves

5cm/2in cinnamon

2 green cardamom pods

1 tsp mustard seeds, ground

1 tbsp salt

Method

- Boil the turnips with the water on a low heat for 15 minutes. Drain and set aside.

- Heat the oil in a saucepan. Fry the garlic and the ginger paste on a low heat till golden brown.
- Add the boiled turnip and all the remaining ingredients. Mix well.
- Cook the mixture until the oil separates.
- Cool and transfer to a clean, dry jar.

NOTE: *This can be stored in a refrigerator for a month.*

Sweet Mango Pickle

Ingredients

500g/1lb 2oz unripe mangoes, peeled and finely sliced

Salt to taste

1 tsp turmeric

120ml/4fl oz refined vegetable oil

2 cloves

2.5cm/1in cinnamon

6 black peppercorns

1 tsp chilli powder

250g/9oz grated jaggery*

5cm/2in root ginger, finely sliced

12 garlic cloves, finely sliced

Method

- Rub the mango slices with the salt and turmeric. Set aside for an hour.
- Squeeze out water by pressing the mango slices between your palms. Set aside.
- Heat the oil in a saucepan. Add the cloves, cinnamon and peppercorns.
- Let them splutter for 15 seconds. Add the mango slices and mix well.

- Add the chilli powder, jaggery, ginger and garlic. Mix well and cook over a low heat till the jaggery melts into a thick syrup.
- Allow the pickle to cool. Store in a dry, clean jar and keep aside for a day.

NOTE: *This can be stored in the refrigerator for a month.*

Carrot Pickle

Ingredients

6½ tbsp refined vegetable oil

1 tsp mustard seeds

1 tsp fenugreek seeds

½ tsp asafoetida

1 tsp turmeric

2 tsp chilli powder

Salt to taste

250g/9oz carrots, thinly sliced

Method

- Heat the oil in a saucepan. Add the mustard seeds, fenugreek seeds, asafoetida, turmeric, chilli powder and the salt. Fry on a low heat for 15 seconds.
- Allow the mixture to cool. Pour over the carrot slices and let stand for 2-3 hours.
- Store in a clean, dry jar.

NOTE: *This can be stored in the refrigerator for a week.*

Green Coconut Chutney

Ingredients

200g/7oz coriander leaves

100g/3½oz grated fresh coconut

2 green chillies

8 garlic cloves

Salt to taste

60ml/2fl oz water

Method

- Grind all the ingredients together. Store in a clean, dry jar.

NOTE: *This can be stored in the refrigerator for 2-3 days.*

Mint Chutney

Ingredients

100g/3½oz fresh mint leaves

1 large onion

3 green chillies

8 garlic cloves

Salt to taste

1 tbsp water

Method

- Grind all the ingredients together. Store in a clean, dry jar for 2-3 days.

Peanut Chutney

Ingredients

250g/9oz roasted peanuts

1 tsp chilli powder

2 tsp sugar

Salt to taste

Method

- Grind all the ingredients together. Store in a clean, dry jar for 10 days.

Papaya Chutney

Ingredients

1 tsp salt

2 tsp sugar

200g/7oz grated unripe papaya

2 tbsp refined vegetable oil

1 tsp cumin seeds

8 curry leaves

3 green chillies, slit lengthways

½ tsp turmeric

Method

- Mix the salt and the sugar with the grated papaya. Set aside.
- Heat the oil in a saucepan. Add the cumin seeds, curry leaves, green chillies and turmeric. Let them splutter for 15 seconds.
- Pour this over the grated papaya mixture. Mix well.
- Allow the mixture to cool and then store in a clean, dry jar.

NOTE: *This can be stored in the refrigerator for a week.*

Sweet & Sour Mango Pickle

Ingredients

500g/1lb 2oz unripe mangoes, peeled and chopped into 5cm/2in strips

Salt to taste

125g/4½oz mustard seeds, coarsely ground

3 tbsp water

180g/6½oz grated jaggery*

1 tsp chilli powder

1½ tbsp refined vegetable oil

1 tsp mustard seeds

½ tsp asafoetida

½ tsp turmeric

Method

- Rub the mango slices with salt. Set aside.
- Mix the ground mustard with half a tsp of salt and the water.
- Mix this well with the mango slices, along with the jaggery and chilli powder.
- Heat the oil in a saucepan. Add the mustard seeds, asafoetida and turmeric. Let them splutter for 15 seconds.

- Remove from the heat and pour this oil over the mango mixture. Mix thoroughly.
- Allow to cool and store in a clean, dry jar.

NOTE: *This can be stored in the refrigerator for a month.*

Aubergine Pickle

Ingredients

120ml/4fl oz refined vegetable oil

1 tsp mustard seeds

1 tsp fenugreek seeds

2 tsp ground cumin

2.5cm/1in root ginger, finely chopped

12 garlic cloves, finely chopped

4 green chillies, finely chopped

500g/1lb 2oz aubergine, chopped into 2.5cm/1in pieces

125g/4½oz sugar

120ml/4fl oz malt vinegar

Salt to taste

Method

- Heat the oil in a saucepan. Add the mustard seeds, fenugreek seeds and ground cumin.
- Let them splutter for 15 seconds. Add the ginger, garlic and green chillies. Fry on a low heat for a minute.
- Add the aubergine pieces. Mix well to coat with the oil. Cook for 3-4 minutes on a medium heat, stirring well.
- Add the sugar, vinegar and the salt. Cook over a low heat till the aubergine pieces become soft. Allow any extra liquid to evaporate.
- Remove from the heat and cool.
- Store in a clean, dry jar.

NOTE: *This can be stored in the refrigerator for a month.*

Curry Leaves Dry Pickle

Ingredients

25g/scant 1oz curry leaves, dry roasted

250g/9oz kaala chana*, roasted

1 tbsp sugar

8 dry red chillies

Salt to taste

Method

- Dry grind all the ingredients together.
- Store in a clean, dry jar.

NOTE: *This can be stored in the refrigerator for a month.*

Tomato Pickle

Ingredients

240ml/6fl oz refined vegetable oil

1 tsp mustard seeds

¼ tsp fenugreek seeds

1 tsp cumin seeds

½ tsp turmeric

8 curry leaves

2 tsp ginger paste

2 tsp garlic paste

2 red chillies, slit lengthways

4 tomatoes, blanched, skinned and chopped

250ml/8fl oz malt vinegar

250g/9oz sugar

Salt to taste

Method

- Heat the oil in a saucepan. Add the mustard seeds, fenugreek seeds, cumin seeds, turmeric, curry leaves, ginger paste, garlic paste and the red chillies. Fry for 30 seconds.
- Add the tomatoes. Mix well.
- Add the vinegar, sugar and salt. Cook on a low heat for 20 minutes.
- Remove from the heat and allow the mixture to cool. Store in clean, dry jar.

NOTE: *This can be stored in the refrigerator for a month.*

Hot Lime Pickle

Ingredients

60g/2oz turmeric

125g/4½oz chilli powder

1 tsp fenugreek seeds

250g/9oz coarse salt

25 limes, each cut into 8 pieces

Juice of 10 lemons

Method

- Add the turmeric, chilli powder, fenugreek seeds and salt to the limes. Mix thoroughly. Transfer to a clean, dry jar.
- Pour the lemon juice over this mixture.
- Seal and set aside in a cool, dry place. Stir the contents every third day for 15 days.

NOTE: *This can be stored in the refrigerator for a month.*

Hot & Sweet Mango Chutney

Ingredients

60ml/2fl oz malt vinegar

3-4 dry red chillies, broken into bits

6 cloves

6 black peppercorns

1 tsp cumin seeds

½ tsp kalonji seeds*

250g/9oz sugar

Salt to taste

500g/1lb 2oz unripe mangoes, peeled and diced

5cm/2in root ginger, finely sliced

10 garlic cloves, finely sliced

Method

- In a deep saucepan, heat the vinegar with the chillies, cloves, peppercorns, cumin seeds, kalonji seeds, sugar and salt.
- Simmer for 15 minutes.
- Add the mango pieces, ginger and garlic.
- Simmer till the mango pieces become mushy and most of the vinegar evaporates.
- Cool the mixture and transfer into a clean, dry jar.
- Refrigerate for 2 days before serving.

NOTE: *This can be stored in a refrigerator for a month.*

Jaggery & Date Chutney

Ingredients

4 tbsp tamarind paste

50g/1¾oz jaggery*

8 dates

240ml/6fl oz water

1 tsp chilli powder

1 tsp ground cumin*

¼ tsp dry ginger powder

½ tbsp black salt

Method

- Mix the tamarind paste, jaggery and dates with the water. Set aside for an hour.
- Transfer the mixture to a saucepan and cook for 5-10 minutes on a low heat.
- Add the chilli powder, ground cumin, dry ginger powder and black salt.
- Mix well and cook for another minute.
- Remove from the heat and cool.

NOTE: *This can be stored in the refrigerator for a month.*

Sour Green Mango Pickle

Ingredients

1kg/2¼lb unripe mangoes

1 tbsp fenugreek seeds

1 tbsp fennel seeds

10g/¼oz kalonji seeds*

2 tsp mustard seeds

500ml/16fl oz mustard oil

For the spice mixture:

125g/4½oz chilli powder

2 tsp cumin seeds

2 tsp turmeric

½ tsp asafoetida

Salt to taste

Method

- Chop the mangoes into 2.5cm/1in pieces and pat them dry with a towel.
- Grind all the ingredients for the spice mixture together.
- To this mixture, add the fenugreek seeds, fennel seeds, kalonji seeds, mustard seeds and the mustard oil. Mix well to make a paste.

- Add the dried mango pieces to the paste. Mix well. Cook this mixture in a saucepan on a low heat for 20 minutes.
- Transfer the pickle into a dry jar.

NOTE: *This pickle can be stored in the refrigerator for a month.*

Coconut Chutney

Ingredients

200g/7oz fresh coconut, grated

8 garlic cloves

6 dry red chillies

1½ tsp tamarind paste

Salt to taste

60ml/2fl oz water

Method

- Grind all the ingredients together.
- Store in a clean, dry jar.

NOTE: *This can be stored in the refrigerator for 2-3 days.*

Mango & Chickpea Pickle

Ingredients

500g/1lb 2oz unripe, unpeeled mangoes

1 tbsp mustard seeds

2 tbsp fenugreek seeds

1 tbsp chilli powder

½ tbsp turmeric

1 tsp asafoetida

Salt to taste

60g/2oz canned chickpeas

500ml/16fl oz refined vegetable oil

Method

- Chop the mangoes into 2.5cm/1in pieces and pat dry with a towel.
- Grind the mustard seeds, fenugreek seeds, chilli powder, turmeric, asafoetida and salt together. Add this to the mango pieces.
- Add the chickpeas and the oil. Cook the mixture in a saucepan on a low heat for 30 minutes.
- Transfer the mixture to a clean, dry porcelain jar.

NOTE: *This can be stored in the refrigerator for a month.*

Dry Garlic Chutney

Ingredients

Salt to taste

2 tsp tamarind paste

For the spice mixture:

20 garlic cloves

200g/7oz desiccated coconut

1 tbsp cumin seeds

2 tbsp sesame seeds

5 dry red chillies

60g/2oz peanuts

Method

- Dry roast all the ingredients for the spice mixture. Coarsely grind them along with the salt.
- Add this mixture to the tamarind paste. Mix thoroughly.
- Store in an airtight container and use when required.

NOTE: *This can be stored in the refrigerator for a fortnight.*

Gooseberry Pickle

(Suitable for making only during summer)

Ingredients

2 tbsp mustard oil

1 tsp fennel seeds

1½ tsp mustard seeds, ground

3 cloves

2.5cm/1in cinnamon

8 black peppercorns, ground

1 tsp turmeric

½ tsp chilli powder

Salt to taste

250g/9oz gooseberries, de-seeded and quartered

Method

- Heat the oil in a saucepan. Add all the ingredients, except the gooseberries. Let them splutter for 15 seconds.
- Pour this oil over the gooseberries. Mix thoroughly.
- Transfer the mixture to a clean jar with a tight lid. Keep in a warm place for a week. Shake regularly and place in the sun whenever possible. Make sure that the gooseberries are always immersed in oil.

NOTE: *This can be stored in the refrigerator for a month.*

Mixed Fruit Chutney

Ingredients

2.5cm/1in root ginger, thinly sliced

8 garlic cloves, thinly sliced

60g/2oz plums, stoned and chopped

60g/2oz apricots, stoned and chopped

1 tbsp raisins

2 apples, cored and chopped

250g/9oz brown sugar

240ml/8fl oz malt vinegar

1 tsp garam masala

1 tsp chilli powder

½ tsp caraway seeds

Salt to taste

Method

- Mix all the ingredients together. Cook in a saucepan over a low heat for 10 minutes. Cool and store in a clean, dry jar.

NOTE: *This can be stored in a refrigerator for a month.*

Sweet Cauliflower Pickle

Ingredients

12 garlic cloves

5cm/2in root ginger

2 tbsp mustard oil

2 tbsp brown sugar

120ml/4fl oz malt vinegar

1 tsp mustard seeds, ground

1 tbsp salt

1 tsp chilli powder

1 tsp turmeric

1 tsp garam masala

500g/1lb 2oz cauliflower, steamed and chopped into small pieces

Method

- Pound the garlic and ginger together.
- Heat the oil in a saucepan. Fry this mixture on a low heat till golden brown. Set aside.
- Mix the sugar and vinegar in another saucepan. Cook for 10 minutes on a low heat till thick. Set aside to cool for 5 minutes.

- To the sugar-vinegar mixture, add the fried ginger-garlic mixture and all the remaining ingredients.
- Mix thoroughly. Transfer to an airtight jar. Set aside for a week.

NOTE: *This can be stored in the refrigerator for a month.*

Vinegar Chillies

Ingredients

Salt to taste

250ml/8fl oz white vinegar

25 whole green chillies

Method

- Add the salt to the vinegar. Mix well.
- Pour this mixture over the chillies and transfer them to a clean, dry jar.
- Set aside for 4-5 hours.

NOTE: *This can be stored in the refrigerator for a week.*

Cucumber Pickle

Ingredients

250g/9oz unpeeled cucumber, sliced

Salt to taste

60ml/2fl oz white vinegar

¼ tsp chilli powder

¼ tsp black peppercorns

½ tsp mustard seeds

¼ tsp ground cinnamon

¼ tsp ground cloves

1 tsp sugar

Method

- Rub the cucumber slices with salt and let them stand for 3-4 hours. Drain the excess moisture and set aside.
- Boil the vinegar with the chilli powder, peppercorns, mustard seeds, ground cinnamon, ground cloves and sugar in a saucepan on a low heat for 10 minutes.
- Add the cucumber pieces and simmer for 5 minutes.
- Remove from the heat and allow the pickle to cool completely.
- Store in a clean, dry jar.

NOTE: *This can be stored in the refrigerator for a fortnight.*

Hot Mango Pickle

Ingredients

3 unripe, unpeeled mangoes, chopped into small pieces

1½ tbsp salt

1 tbsp turmeric

500ml/16fl oz refined vegetable oil

2 tsp mustard seeds

1 tsp asafoetida

1 tbsp chilli powder

Method

- Rub the mango pieces with the salt and turmeric. Set aside for 5-6 hours.
- Squeeze out the water from the mango pieces. Leave them to dry for another hour.
- Heat the oil in a saucepan. Add the mustard seeds, asafoetida and chilli powder. Let them splutter for 15 seconds.
- Pour this oil mixture over the mango pieces. The oil should cover the mango pieces.
- Store in a dry jar and set aside for 2-3 days.

NOTE: *This can be stored in the refrigerator for a month.*

Cucumber Salad

Ingredients

4 cucumbers, peeled and finely chopped

25g/scant 1oz coriander leaves, finely chopped

180g/6½oz peanuts, coarsely pounded

2 green chillies, coarsely chopped

1 tsp sugar (optional)

1 tsp lemon juice

Salt to taste

Method

- Mix all the ingredients together.
- Serve chilled.

Potato Salad

Serves 4

Ingredients

4 large potatoes, diced and boiled

1 large onion, finely chopped

1 green chilli, finely chopped

1 tbsp coriander leaves, finely chopped

2 tsp cumin seeds, dry roasted and ground

3 tsp lemon juice

Salt to taste

Method

- Mix all the ingredients together.
- Serve chilled.

Koshimbir

Ingredients

4 tomatoes, finely chopped

2 large onions, finely chopped

10g/¼oz coriander leaves, finely chopped

50g/1¾oz roasted peanuts, coarsely pounded

½ tsp sugar (optional)

1 tsp lemon juice

Salt to taste

Method

- Mix all the ingredients together.
- Serve chilled.

Green Pepper Salad

Serves 4

Ingredients

2 green peppers, roughly chopped

50g/1¾oz pineapple, roughly chopped

50g/1¾oz spring onions, finely chopped

25g/scant 1oz coriander leaves, finely chopped

Freshly ground black pepper to taste

2 tsp lemon juice

Salt to taste

Method

- Mix all the ingredients together.
- Serve chilled.

Mint Pasta Salad

Serves 4

Ingredients

100g/3½oz cooked penne pasta

25g/scant 1oz mint leaves, finely chopped

1 large potato, diced and boiled

50g/1¾oz spring onions, finely chopped

3 tsp ground cumin, dry roasted

½ tsp ground black pepper

1 tbsp lemon juice

Salt to taste

Method

- Mix all the ingredients together.
- Serve chilled.

Mushroom Salad

Serves 4

Ingredients

300g/10oz mushrooms

50g/1¾oz spring onions, thinly sliced

1 red or yellow pepper, thinly sliced

3 tsp ground cumin, dry roasted

1 tbsp lemon juice

Salt to taste

Method

- Soak the mushrooms in hot water for 5 minutes. Drain and slice.
- Mix with the remaining ingredients. Serve chilled.

Egg Salad

Serves 4

Ingredients

1 large onion, finely chopped

10g/¼oz coriander leaves, chopped

2 green chillies, finely chopped

2 tsp lemon juice

1 tsp chaat masala*

Salt to taste

6 hard-boiled eggs, diced

Method

- Mix all the ingredients, except the eggs, together.
- Add the eggs. Mix gently. Serve.

Mixed Fruit Salad

Serves 4

Ingredients

1 apple, diced

50g/1¾oz pineapple, diced

1 pear, diced

6 strawberries, coarsely chopped

2 tsp chaat masala*

2 tsp lemon juice

Salt to taste

Sugar to taste

Method

- Mix all the ingredients together.
- Serve chilled.

Carrot Salad

Serves 4

Ingredients

2 large carrots, grated

3 tbsp peanuts, coarsely powdered

3 green chillies, finely chopped

1 tsp sugar

2 tsp lemon juice

Ground black pepper to taste

1 tbsp coriander leaves, chopped

Salt to taste

Method

- Mix all the ingredients together.
- Serve chilled.

Sprouted Beans Salad

Serves 4

Ingredients

500g/1lb 2oz mung bean sprouts, steamed

1 tomato, finely chopped

2 green chillies, finely chopped

1 large onion, finely chopped

1 tsp sugar

10g/¼oz coriander leaves, chopped

Salt to taste

Method

- Mix all the ingredients together.
- Serve chilled.

Kaala Chana & Peanut Salad

Serves 4

Ingredients

250g/9oz kaala chana*, boiled

250g/9oz roasted peanuts

1 tbsp coriander leaves, finely chopped

1 large onion, finely grated

1 tsp chaat masala*

Juice of 1 lemon

2 green chillies, finely chopped

Salt to taste

Method

- Mix all the ingredients together.
- Serve chilled.

Mixed Salad

Serves 4

Ingredients

125g/4½oz cabbage, grated

1 tomato, finely chopped

1 cucumber, finely chopped

1 carrot, grated

2 tsp chaat masala*

2 tsp lemon juice

Salt to taste

Method

- Mix all the ingredients together.
- Serve chilled.

Cabbage & Pomegranate Salad

Serves 4

Ingredients

Salt to taste

150g/5½oz grated cabbage

200g/7oz pomegranate seeds

1 tbsp coriander leaves, finely chopped

1 tsp chaat masala*

2 tsp refined vegetable oil

1 tsp cumin seeds

Method

- Sprinkle the salt on top of the cabbage and set aside for 30 minutes. Squeeze out water from the cabbage by pressing it between your palms
- Add the pomegranate seeds, coriander and chaat masala. Set aside.
- Heat the oil in a saucepan. Add the cumin seeds. Let them splutter for 15 seconds. Pour this over the cabbage mixture. Serve chilled.

Fish Salad

Serves 4

Ingredients

½ tsp chilli powder

¾ tsp turmeric

1 tsp tamarind paste

1 tsp ginger paste

1 tsp garlic paste

Salt to taste

500g/1lb 2oz boneless fish or fillets, chopped into 5cm/2in pieces

2 tbsp refined vegetable oil

1 large onion, finely sliced

2 tbsp coriander leaves, finely chopped

1 tbsp lemon juice

1 tsp chaat masala*

2 green chillies, finely chopped

Method

- Mix the chilli powder, turmeric, tamarind paste, ginger paste, garlic paste and salt together. Marinate the fish with the mixture for 30 minutes.
- Heat the oil in a saucepan. Shallow fry the fish on a medium heat till it is cooked on both sides. Drain on absorbent paper. Allow to cool, then roughly shred the fish.
- Mix thoroughly with all the remaining ingredients. Serve chilled.

Spicy Chicken Salad

Serves 4

Ingredients

600g/1lb 5oz skinned boneless chicken, cut into 2.5cm/1in pieces

2 large onions, thinly sliced

3 green chillies, slit lengthwise

1 tsp lemon juice

25g/scant 1oz coriander leaves, finely chopped

Salt to taste

For the marinade:

½ tsp chilli powder

1 tsp freshly ground black pepper

½ tsp turmeric

60ml/2fl oz sour cream

1 tsp ginger paste

1 tsp garlic paste

1 tsp ground coriander

1 tsp ground cumin

1 tsp lemon juice

Method

- Mix the marinade ingredients together. Marinate the chicken pieces with this mixture for 30 minutes.
- Grill the chicken for 15 minutes.
- Add the remaining ingredients. Mix well. Serve chilled.

Watermelon Salad

Serves 4

Ingredients

½ watermelon

8 garlic cloves, finely chopped

1 tbsp coriander leaves, finely chopped

25g/scant 1oz spring onion, finely chopped

Juice of 1 lemon

Salt to taste

Method

- Scoop out the flesh of the watermelon. Carefully deseed and dice. Do not discard the shell.
- Mix the watermelon pieces with the garlic, coriander leaves, spring onion, lemon juice and salt.
- Place this mixture back into the shell. Serve chilled.

Cabbage Salad

Serves 4

Ingredients

50g/1¾oz sprouted mung beans

500g/1lb 2oz cabbage, finely grated

25g/scant 1oz fresh coconut, grated

1 tbsp coriander leaves, finely chopped

2 tsp sugar

1 tbsp lemon juice

Salt to taste

2 tsp refined vegetable oil

½ tsp mustard seeds

8 curry leaves

¼ tsp turmeric

3 green chillies, slit lengthways

Method

- In a bowl, mix the mung beans with the cabbage, coconut, coriander leaves, sugar, lemon juice and salt. Set aside.
- Heat the oil in a saucepan. Add the mustard seeds, curry leaves, turmeric and green chillies. Let them splutter for 15 seconds. Pour this over the cabbage mixture. Mix thoroughly.
- Serve chilled.

French Bean Salad

Serves 4

Ingredients

Salt to taste

250g/9oz French beans, finely chopped

1 large onion, finely chopped

1 tsp lemon juice

1 tsp honey

1 tsp ground cumin, dry roasted

1 tbsp coriander leaves, finely chopped

1 tbsp fresh coconut, grated

Method

- Add the salt to the beans and steam them, keeping them slightly crunchy.
- Mix with all the other ingredients in a bowl.
- Serve at room temperature.

Water Chestnut Salad

Ingredients

1 tbsp refined vegetable oil

½ tsp ginger paste

½ tsp garlic paste

1 red pepper, julienned

1 yellow pepper, julienned

1 green pepper, julienned

50g/1¾oz spring onions, finely chopped

4 green chillies, slit lengthwise

300g/10oz water chestnuts, par-boiled and quartered

Salt to taste

¾ tsp ground black pepper

2 tsp soy sauce

Method

- Heat the oil in a saucepan. Add the ginger paste and garlic paste. Fry for a few seconds on a medium heat.
- Add all the remaining ingredients. Sauté for 30 seconds. Serve immediately.

NOTE: *The salad should be crunchy when it is served.*

Vermicelli & Corn Salad

Serves 4

Ingredients

1 tsp refined vegetable oil

½ tsp cumin seeds

1 large onion, finely chopped

100g/3½oz vermicelli, boiled and drained

200g/7oz boiled corn

2 tbsp coriander leaves, chopped

2 tsp lemon juice

1 tsp ground cumin, dry roasted

2 green chillies, finely chopped

Method

- Heat the oil in a saucepan. Add the cumin seeds. Let them splutter for 15 seconds. Add the onion and fry for a few seconds on a medium heat.
- Add all the remaining ingredients. Toss well. Serve immediately.

Rice Salad

Serves 6

Ingredients

100g/3½oz steamed basmati rice (see here)

125g/4½oz boiled peas

50g/1¾oz cauliflower florets, boiled

50g/1¾oz carrots, diced and boiled

60g/2oz roasted peanuts

1 tbsp lemon juice

1 tsp caster sugar

Salt to taste

2 tsp refined vegetable oil

1 tsp cumin seeds

5-6 curry leaves, roughly torn

2 tbsp coriander leaves, finely chopped

Method

- Mix the rice, peas, cauliflower florets, carrots, peanuts, lemon juice, sugar and salt together in a bowl. Set aside.
- Heat the oil in a saucepan. Add the cumin seeds and curry leaves. Let them splutter for 15 seconds.
- Pour this over the rice mixture. Toss lightly.
- Garnish with the coriander leaves. Serve immediately.

Daikon Salad

Ingredients

2 daikons, grated

Salt to taste

2 tsp sugar

2 tsp refined vegetable oil

1 tsp mustard seeds

8 curry leaves

2 green chillies, slit lengthways

1 tbsp coriander leaves, finely chopped

½ tbsp lemon juice

Method

- In a bowl, mix the daikon with the salt and sugar. Set aside.
- Heat the oil in a saucepan. Add the mustard seeds, curry leaves and green chillies. Let them splutter for 15 seconds.
- Pour this oil over the daikon mixture. Add the coriander leaves and lemon juice. Mix thoroughly. Serve chilled.

Peanut & Chickpea Salad

Serves 4

Ingredients

125g/4½oz peanuts

75g/2½oz chickpeas, soaked for 2 hours

60g/2oz kaala chana*, soaked for 2 hours

750ml/1¼fl oz water

1 large green pepper, cored, deseeded and finely chopped

50g/1¾oz coriander leaves, finely chopped

1 large tomato, finely chopped

1 large onion, finely chopped

2 green chillies, finely chopped

2 tsp lemon juice

2 tsp chaat masala*

Salt to taste

Method

- In a saucepan, boil the peanuts, chickpeas and kaala chana with the water on a high heat for 45 minutes.
- Transfer to a bowl. Add the remaining ingredients and mix well.
- Serve chilled.

Rajma Salad

(Kidney Bean Salad)

Serves 4

Ingredients

Salt to taste

2 tbsp malt vinegar

600g/1lb 5oz canned kidney beans

1 large onion, finely chopped

1 tomato, finely chopped

5 cloves

2 green chillies, finely chopped

1 tbsp coriander leaves, finely chopped

Method

- Sprinkle salt and vinegar on top of the kidney beans. Mix well and set aside for 10 minutes.
- Add the remaining ingredients. Mix thoroughly and serve chilled.

Beetroot Salad

Serves 4

Ingredients

250g/9oz beetroot, boiled and grated

125g/4½oz peanuts, coarsely pounded

2 tsp lemon juice

1 tbsp coriander leaves, finely chopped

Salt to taste

2 tsp refined vegetable oil

1 tsp cumin seeds

2 green chillies, slit lengthways

Method

- In a bowl, mix the beetroot, peanuts, lemon juice, coriander leaves and salt. Set aside.
- Heat the oil in a saucepan. Add the cumin seeds and slit green chillies. Let them splutter for 15 seconds.
- Pour this mixture over the beetroot mixture. Mix well.
- Serve chilled.

Paneer Salad

Serves 4

Ingredients

1 green pepper, diced

1 large onion, finely chopped

125g/4½oz pomegranate seeds

3 tsp chaat masala*

10g/¼oz coriander leaves, finely chopped

2 tsp lemon juice

Salt to taste

500g/1lb 2oz paneer*,

diced

Method

- In a bowl, mix all the ingredients thoroughly, except the paneer.
- Add the paneer pieces gently, making sure they do not crumble. Mix carefully.
- Serve chilled.

Corn Salad

Serves 24

Ingredients

2 tsp refined vegetable oil

½ tsp cumin seeds

1 large onion, finely chopped

2 green chillies, finely chopped

1 tomato, finely chopped

400g/14oz boiled corn kernels

Salt to taste

2 tsp lemon juice

1 tsp chaat masala*

1 tbsp coriander leaves, finely chopped

Method

- Heat the oil in a saucepan. Add the cumin seeds. Let them splutter for 15 seconds.
- Add the onion and fry for a minute.
- Add the chillies, tomato, corn and salt. Cook for a minute, stirring continuously.
- Add the lemon juice, chaat masala and coriander leaves.
- Serve at room temperature.

Stir-Fried Salad

Ingredients

2 tsp refined vegetable oil

100g/3½oz mushrooms, sliced

100g/3½oz baby corn, sliced lengthwise

1 green pepper, cored, deseeded and sliced

½ tsp ground black pepper

2 green chillies, slit lengthways

Salt to taste

1 tomato, finely sliced

1 tsp lemon juice

Method

- Heat the oil in a saucepan. Add the mushrooms, baby corn and green pepper. Stir-fry on a high heat for 2 minutes.
- Add the remaining ingredients. Cook for another minute on a medium heat. Serve warm.

Spinach Salad

Serves 4

Ingredients

200g/7oz spinach, chopped

1.5 litres/2¾ pints salted hot water

1½ tbsp clear honey

½ tbsp roasted sesame seeds

½ tbsp lemon juice

Salt to taste

Method

- Soak the spinach in the water for 2 minutes and drain completely.
- Add all the remaining ingredients to the spinach. Mix well.
- Serve chilled.

Prawn Salad

Serves 4

Ingredients

250g/9oz prawns, shelled and de-veined

Salt to taste

1 tbsp lemon juice

750 ml/1¼fl oz water

50g/1¾oz spring onions, finely chopped

10g/¼oz coriander leaves, finely chopped

3 tsp chaat masala*

2 green chillies, finely chopped

1 tomato, finely chopped

1 green pepper, finely chopped

Method

- Boil the prawns in a saucepan with the salt, lemon juice and water on a medium heat for 10 minutes. Drain and cool.
- Mix thoroughly with all the other ingredients in a bowl.
- Serve chilled.

Pineapple & Honey Raita

Serves 4

Ingredients

250g/9oz pineapple, diced

85g/3oz mixed nuts (cashew nuts, pistachios and walnuts)

1 tsp honey

450g/1lb yoghurt

Salt to taste

Method

- Mix all the ingredients together in a bowl.
- Serve chilled.

Mango Raita

Serves 4

Ingredients

450g/1lb ripe mangoes, peeled and diced

450g/1lb yoghurt

¼ tsp saffron, soaked in 1 tbsp milk

Salt to taste

Method

- Mix all the ingredients together in a bowl.
- Serve chilled.

Apple Walnut Raita

Serves 4

Ingredients

2 apples, cored and diced

85g/3oz walnuts, chopped

350g/12oz yoghurt

Salt to taste

Method

- Mix all the ingredients together in a bowl.
- Serve chilled.

Bottle Gourd Raita

Serves 4

Ingredients

1 bottle gourd*, peeled and grated

350g/12oz yoghurt

½ tsp ground black pepper

1 tbsp coriander leaves, finely chopped

Salt to taste

Method

- Steam the bottle gourd till soft.
- Squeeze out the excess water and mix with the remaining ingredients. Serve chilled.

Cucumber Raita

Serves 4

Ingredients

1 large cucumber, grated

450g/1lb yoghurt

2 green chillies, slit lengthways

1 tbsp ready-made mustard

Salt to taste

Method

- Squeeze out the excess water from the cucumber.
- Add all the remaining ingredients. Mix well. Serve chilled.

Carrot Raita

Serves 4

Ingredients

2 large carrots, finely grated

450g/1lb yoghurt

2 green chillies, slit lengthways

2 tbsp roasted peanuts

1 tsp sugar (optional)

Salt to taste

Method

- Mix all the ingredients well in a bowl. Serve chilled.

Mustard Raita

Serves 4

Ingredients

450g/1lb yoghurt

2 tsp ground mustard

1 green chilli, finely chopped

½ tsp ground black pepper

Salt to taste

Method

- In a bowl, whisk the yoghurt with all the other ingredients.
- Serve chilled.

Spring Onion Raita

Serves 4

Ingredients

100g/3½oz spring onions, chopped

350g/12oz yoghurt

1 tbsp coriander leaves, finely chopped

1 green chilli, finely chopped

Salt to taste

Method

- Mix all the ingredients well in a bowl.
- Serve chilled.

Pineapple Raita

Serves 4

Ingredients

100g/3½oz canned pineapple pieces, diced

450g/1lb yoghurt

Salt to taste

Method

- Mix all the ingredients well in a bowl.
- Serve chilled.

Potato Raita

Serves 4

Ingredients

2 large potatoes, boiled and diced

450g/1lb yoghurt

1 tsp chaat masala*

1 tbsp coriander leaves, chopped

1 small onion, finely grated (optional)

Salt to taste

Method

- Mix all the ingredients well in a bowl. Serve chilled.

Spinach Raita

Serves 4

Ingredients

100g/3½oz spinach leaves, finely chopped

250ml/8fl oz hot water

450g/1lb Greek yoghurt

Pinch of chaat masala*

2 green chillies, slit lengthways

Salt to taste

Method

- Soak the spinach leaves in the hot water for 5 minutes. Drain out the water and mix the spinach with the remaining ingredients. Serve chilled.

Mixed Fruit Raita

Serves 4

Ingredients

1 apple, cored and diced

20 green grapes

1 orange, de-seeded and diced

450g/1lb yoghurt

1 tsp chaat masala*

Salt to taste

Method

- Mix all the ingredients well in a bowl. Serve chilled.

Banana Raita

Ingredients

2 large ripe bananas, peeled and sliced

350g/12oz yoghurt

2 tsp caster sugar

¼ tsp grated nutmeg

¼ tsp green cardamom seeds, ground

A pinch of salt

Method

- Mix all the ingredients well in a bowl. Serve chilled.

Guava Raita

Serves 4

Ingredients

1 large ripe guava, peeled and diced

450g/1lb yoghurt

1 tsp ground cumin, dry roasted

1 green chilli, slit lengthways

¼ tsp ground black pepper

1 tsp caster sugar

Salt to taste

Method

- Mix all the ingredients well in a bowl. Serve chilled.

Batter Fried Fish

Serves 4

Ingredients

1kg/2¼lb monkfish, skinned and filleted

½ tsp turmeric

Salt to taste

125g/4½oz besan*

3 tbsp breadcrumbs

½ tsp chilli powder

½ tsp ground black pepper

1 green chilli, chopped

1 tsp ajowan seeds

3 tbsp chopped coriander leaves

500ml/16fl oz water

Refined vegetable oil for deep frying

Method

- Marinate the fish with the turmeric and salt for 30 minutes.

- Mix together the remaining ingredients, except the oil, to form a batter.

- Heat the oil in a pan. Dip the marinated fish in the batter and deep fry on a medium heat till golden brown.

- Drain on absorbent paper and serve hot.

Fish Caldine

(Goan-style Fish)

Serves 4

Ingredients

3 tbsp refined vegetable oil

3 large onions, finely sliced

6 green chillies, slit lengthways

750g/1lb 10oz filleted sea bass, chopped

1 tsp ground cumin

1 tsp turmeric

1 tsp ginger paste

1 tsp garlic paste

360ml/12fl oz coconut milk

2 tsp tamarind paste

Salt to taste

Method

- Heat the oil in a saucepan. Add the onions and fry on a low heat till brown.

- Add the green chillies, fish, ground cumin, turmeric, ginger paste, garlic paste and the coconut milk. Mix well and simmer for 10 minutes.

- Add the tamarind paste and salt. Mix well and simmer for 15 minutes. Serve hot.

Prawn and Egg Curry

Serves 4

Ingredients

3 tbsp refined vegetable oil

2 cloves

2.5cm/1in cinnamon

6 black peppercorns

2 bay leaves

1 large onion, finely chopped

½ tsp turmeric

1 tsp ginger paste

1 tsp garlic paste

1 tsp garam masala

12 large prawns, shelled and de-veined

Salt to taste

200g/7oz tomato purée

120ml/4fl oz water

4 hard-boiled eggs, halved lengthways

Method

- Heat the oil in a saucepan. Add the cloves, cinnamon, peppercorns and bay leaves. Let them splutter for 15 seconds.

- Add the remaining ingredients, except the tomato purée, water and eggs. Sauté on a medium heat for 6-7 minutes. Add the tomato purée and water. Simmer for 10-12 minutes.

- Add the eggs carefully. Simmer for 4-5 minutes. Serve hot.

Fish Molee

(Fish cooked in Basic Simple Curry)

Serves 4

Ingredients

2 tbsp ghee

1 small onion, finely chopped

4 garlic cloves, finely sliced

2.5cm/1in root ginger, finely sliced

6 green chillies, slit lengthways

1 tsp turmeric

Salt to taste

750ml/1¼ pints coconut milk

1kg/2¼lb sea bass, skinned and filleted

Method

- Heat the ghee in a saucepan. Add the onion, garlic, ginger and chillies. Fry on a low heat for 2 minutes. Add the turmeric. Cook for 3-4 minutes.

- Add the salt, coconut milk and fish. Mix well and simmer for 15-20 minutes. Serve hot.

Prawns Bharta

(Prawns cooked in Classic Indian Gravy)

Serves 4

Ingredients

100ml/3½fl oz mustard oil

1 tsp cumin seeds

1 large onion, grated

1 tsp turmeric

1 tsp garam masala

2 tsp ginger paste

2 tsp garlic paste

2 tomatoes, finely chopped

3 green chillies, slit lengthways

750g/1lb 10oz prawns, shelled and de-veined

250ml/8fl oz water

Salt to taste

Method

- Heat the oil in a saucepan. Add the cumin seeds. Let them splutter for 15 seconds. Add the onion and fry on a medium heat till brown.

- Add all the remaining ingredients. Simmer for 15 minutes and serve hot.

Spicy Fish & Vegetables

Serves 4

Ingredients

2 tbsp mustard oil

500g/1lb 2oz lemon sole, skinned and filleted

¼ tsp mustard seeds

¼ tsp fennel seeds

¼ tsp fenugreek seeds

¼ tsp cumin seeds

2 bay leaves

½ tsp turmeric

2 dry red chillies, halved

1 large onion, finely sliced

200g/7oz frozen mixed vegetables

360ml/12fl oz water

Salt to taste

Method

- Heat the oil in a saucepan. Add the fish and shallow fry on a medium heat till golden brown. Flip and repeat. Drain and set aside.

- To the same oil, add the mustard, fennel, fenugreek and cumin seeds, bay leaves, turmeric and red chillies. Fry for 30 seconds.

- Add the onion. Fry on a medium heat for 1 minute. Add the remaining ingredients and the fried fish. Simmer for 30 minutes and serve hot.

Mackerel Cutlet

Serves 4

Ingredients

4 large mackerel, cleaned

Salt to taste

½ tsp turmeric

2 tsp malt vinegar

250ml/8fl oz water

1 tbsp refined vegetable oil plus extra for shallow frying

2 big onions, finely chopped

1 tsp ginger paste

1 tsp garlic paste

1 tomato, finely chopped

1 tsp ground black pepper

1 egg, whisked

10g/¼oz coriander leaves, chopped

3 bread slices, soaked and squeezed

60g/2oz rice flour

Method

- Cook the mackerel in a saucepan with the salt, turmeric, vinegar and water on a medium heat for 15 minutes. De-bone and mash. Set aside.

- Heat 1 tbsp oil in a saucepan. Fry the onions on a low heat till brown.

- Add the ginger paste, garlic paste and tomato. Sauté for 4-5 minutes.

- Add the pepper and salt and remove from the heat. Mix with the mashed fish, egg, coriander leaves and bread. Knead and shape into 8 cutlets.

- Heat the oil in a frying pan. Roll the cutlets in the rice flour and shallow fry on a medium heat for 4-5 minutes. Flip and repeat. Serve hot.

Tandoori Crab

Serves 4

Ingredients

2 tsp ginger paste

2 tsp garlic paste

2 tsp garam masala

1 tbsp lemon juice

125g/4½oz Greek yoghurt

Salt to taste

4 crabs, cleaned

1 tbsp refined vegetable oil

Method

- Mix all ingredients together except the crabs and oil. Marinate the crabs with this mixture for 3-4 hours.
- Brush the marinated crab with the oil. Grill for 10-15 minutes. Serve hot.

Stuffed Fish

Ingredients

2 tbsp refined vegetable oil plus extra for shallow frying

1 large onion, finely minced

1 large tomato, finely chopped

1 tsp ginger paste

1 tsp garlic paste

1 tsp ground coriander

1 tsp ground cumin

Salt to taste

1 tsp turmeric

2 tbsp malt vinegar

1kg/2¼lb salmon, slit at the belly

25g/scant 1oz breadcrumbs

Method

- Heat 2 tbsp of the oil in a saucepan. Add the onion and fry on a low heat till brown. Add the remaining ingredients, except the vinegar, fish and breadcrumbs. Sauté for 5 minutes.
- Add the vinegar. Simmer for 5 minutes. Stuff the fish with the mixture.
- Heat the remaining oil in a frying pan. Roll the fish in the breadcrumbs and shallow fry on a medium heat till golden brown. Flip and repeat. Serve hot.

Prawn & Cauliflower Curry

Serves 4

Ingredients

10 tbsp refined vegetable oil

1 large onion, finely chopped

¾ tsp turmeric

250g/9oz prawns, shelled and de-veined

200g/7oz cauliflower florets

Salt to taste

For the spice mixture:

1 tbsp coriander seeds

1 tbsp garam masala

5 red chillies

2.5cm/1in root ginger

8 garlic cloves

60g/2oz fresh coconut

Method

- Heat half the oil in a frying pan. Add the spice mixture ingredients and fry on a medium heat for 5 minutes. Grind to a thick paste. Set aside.
- Heat the remaining oil in a saucepan. Fry the onion on a medium heat till translucent. Add all the remaining ingredients and the spice paste.
- Simmer for 15-20 minutes, stirring occasionally. Serve hot.

Stir-Fried Clams

Ingredients

500g/1lb 2oz clams, cleaned

6 tbsp refined vegetable oil

2 large onions, finely chopped

1 tsp turmeric

1 tsp garam masala

2 tsp ginger paste

2 tsp garlic paste

10g/¼oz coriander leaves, chopped

6 kokums*

Salt to taste

250ml/8fl oz water

Method

- Steam the clams for 25 minutes. Set aside.
- Heat the oil in a saucepan. Fry the onions on a low heat till brown.
- Add the remaining ingredients, except the water. Sauté for 5-6 minutes.
- Add the steamed clams and the water. Cover with a lid and simmer for 10 minutes. Serve hot.

Lightning Source UK Ltd.
Milton Keynes UK
UKHW021846180521
383961UK00003B/280